he Rough Guide to

HiLDHOOD
LLNesses

CREDITS AND PUBLISHING INFORMATION

Medical advice

While every care has been taken in researching and compiling the medical information in this book, it is in no way intended to replace or supersede professional medical advice. Neither the author nor the publisher may be held responsible for any action or any claim howsoever resulting from the use of this book or any information contained in it. Readers must obtain their own professional medical advice before relying on or otherwise making use of the medical information contained in this book. The Department of Health have offered advice on the factual information within the immunisation section of this book.

Contact details for organisations and website addresses frequently change: those included in this book were correct at the time of publication.

All rights reserved. Copyright © Kaz Cooke 2009
Illustrations copyright © Kaz Cooke 2009
The moral right of the author has been asserted.
This edition first published July 2009 by Rough Guides Ltd:
80 Strand, London WC2R 0RL www.roughguides.com.
This book is based closely on the 'health' and 'immunisation' chapters of *The Rough Guide to Babies and Toddlers* by Kaz Cooke.

ISBN 978-1-84836530-8   1 3 5 7 9 8 6 4 2

Acknowledgement

The Department of Health supported the publication of this book but the individual views expressed are those of the author and do not necessarily reflect official policies.

The Rough Guide to

CHILDHOOD ILLNESSES

CONTENTS

Part 2: immunisation 24

Part 3: childhood diseases & what to do about them 40

Part 4: more info & contacts 50

iNTRODUCTiON: CHiLDReN'S HeaLTH aND CHiLDHOOD iLLNeSSeS

We all want our kids to be happy and well, but the reality is that even generally healthy babies and kids will get sick. Viruses and bacteria (germs) are always lurking about. Some childhood illnesses are minor – sniffles and tummy upsets that come and go quickly with no lasting effects. Babies and children who are getting and "fighting off" illnesses are, in a way, training their immune systems to recognise and prepare to fight off the same illnesses in the future. (Although some annoying illnesses can recur even if you've done battle with them in the past.) This book, based on the health chapter of the *Rough Guide to Babies and Toddlers* and supplemented with updated information, will help you understand and treat your child's illnesses. The experience of kids being sick can range from a few miserable days lurking about in pyjamas and needing lots of cuddles to a scary episode fraught with worry. Knowing how to get the right diagnosis and help with the right treatment can give you peace of mind that you are doing all you can. Everything from the common cold and throwing-up to far more dangerous diseases, such as measles and meningitis, is covered here.

The book also explains how to prevent those more serious illnesses and diseases which used to injure, maim and kill children in the past. Although we don't often hear of these diseases so much, they are still lurking and we still need the protection for our children that, in some cases, only immunisation can provide. In the UK, families can take advantage of the free immunisation programme available to all babies and kids. You may have heard some debate about whether the MMR immunisation jab causes autism. This book is designed to show you that after all the research that has been done and the re-checking of medical histories of millions of children who've been immunised with MMR, it's now clear that childhood immunisation injections – MMR included – do not cause autism. All the details on this and other concerns are discussed here so you can decide for yourself how to best look after your family, based on the best possible information available.

I know I feel better now that my family is fully immunised. It won't stop every illness, or the irregular sniffles, or the occasional day when everyone stays in their pyjamas and stares into the bottom of the "sick bowl". But it means that as a mum, I don't have to worry about most of the really scary stuff, because we've done everything we can to be protected.

Kaz Cooke

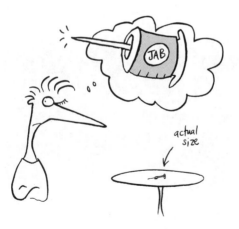

PART 1
getting ill

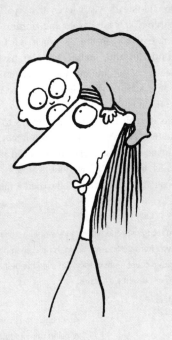

Part 1: getting ill

WHEN CHILDREN get sick

The first six to twelve months of major contact with other kids (siblings or kids at childcare, nursery or school) means it's a germ free-for-all. This is one of the reasons it's so hard for a parent to work outside the home during the child's early years, even if it's part time. Luckily, very few of the things kids are developing immunity against are going to kill them, especially in the UK, where our hospital staff are all generally wonderful and, until recently, we have had universal immunisation (see Part 2 on immunisation). Kids usually get ill suddenly, although after a while you might be able to recognise when they're "fighting off something".

When a kid gets ill their immune system works to develop future protection including developing antibodies (proteins in the blood which fight off invader illnesses). Healthy kids can pick up a minor viral infection, which they fight off without treatment, every couple of months (a head cold, being quiet and "off-colour" – meaning paler – or

---

THE IMMUNE SYSTEM

The immune system recognises and repels many viruses and bacteria you've had before, preventing you from getting sick again. Having an immune system in good shape helps kids recover more quickly. But even the best immune system won't stop all germs or prevent all illnesses.

Good health boosters:

* breastfeeding
* fresh air
* exercise

* enough protein and carbohydrates
* being calm and happy
* fruit and veg

an unidentified rash might be clues). As well as that there are minor sniffles and assorted "tummy bugs" that kids tend to pick up and get rid of over a day or so here and there. If your kid has a chronic or very serious illness, make sure you get all the medical opinions you can and insist on seeing a specialist with the widest possible experience in the area.

What causes illnesses?

Childhood illnesses are usually caused by a virus or bacteria, which are both germs. Viruses are "bugs" that need to live and multiply in cells to survive, so they live in us and reproduce themselves by being passed on to other people, who then get ill and pass them on, and so it goes. Bacteria are little organisms that can live and grow independently (such as germs on a loo seat), with the side effect of infecting people.

When are illnesses contagious?

Illnesses are usually most contagious when the germs are multiplying the fastest. This often happens when you first "catch a bug", before any symptoms appear, and in the first few days of symptoms. Sneezing, vomiting and diarrhoea are really efficient ways of spreading the germs, so while these symptoms continue, whatever the stage of the illness, the bug is probably still contagious. It usually takes three to five days for the incubation of a common cold, meaning from catching it to the start of symptoms. Despite the fact that parents often say "It's not contagious any more", they're often just guessing.

Should kids go back to playgroup, childcare or nursery?

Childcare centres usually say kids with a tummy bug should be kept home until 24 hours after their last vomit or bout of diarrhoea.

Kids should be kept home from group care while they continue to have symptoms of an illness and until they're feeling bouncy again – not only because the bug is still contagious, although that's

WHEN TO CALL AN AMBULANCE FOR A CHILD WITH AN ILLNESS

Ring the general emergency number: 999

Call an ambulance if your child:

★ has a convulsion (a fit).

★ has difficulty with or stops breathing.

★ can't be roused.

★ if they have this combination of symptoms: fever, repeated vomiting, a stiff neck, their eyes are sensitive to light, and they have a spotty rash that starts as red but turns purple and doesn't fade when you press it (these are signs of septicaemia and meningitis), then you need to get your child to a hospital *straight away* – so call an ambulance if you're too stressed to drive safely.

a big issue, especially with more serious illnesses, but because kids with symptoms are almost always below par or even miserable. It's harder for them to get one-on-one care in a childcare centre, even though I know staff do their very best. It isn't fair to the child, and they want to be at home with a parent. Many parents who work outside the home eat up their own annual leave allowance (if they have one) looking after their kids.

When to see a doctor about an illness

Keep the phone number of your GP's surgery near the phone. If the surgery is closed a recorded message should give you the number of your local out-of-hours service, which you can ring for a telephone consultation with a doctor. They may do a home visit, but if they think the problem is really serious they will probably tell you to get to your nearest hospital. My cousin Suze, a paramedic, says "as well as getting better quickly, kids can often deteriorate quickly". She says parents need to keep a careful eye on an ill kid: "It's always suspicious if a child is quieter than usual. It's generally better to have a screaming one than a quiet one."

See or contact a doctor in any of the following situations:

★ Your kid has been in contact with an infectious disease they haven't been immunised against (see Part 2 for details).

★ Fever is accompanied by worrying symptoms such as misery, listlessness, repeated vomiting or an inexplicable rash (see also "When to call an ambulance for a child with an illness", opposite).

★ You're worried because your child seems somehow "not right", too quiet, uninterested in anything or "floppy".

★ Your child develops wheezing.

★ There's unexplained crying that isn't helped by the usual methods, especially in kids who can't tell you what's wrong.

You know your child best so take your own uneasy feelings seriously. All parents have these: some call them "instincts" and act on them, others mistrust them and are unsure whether they're worrying unnecessarily, but they're the same feelings so start calling yours instincts. The only way to check them out is to take your child to a doctor. Even if nothing is revealed, keep on trusting your instincts – you may need to try another doctor or the kid may have just beaten a bug.

Sometimes the only symptom of a kid's illness is listlessness, whingeing and a pressing need to be right next to mum or dad, or at least in the same room. A nurse I know always tested her post-toddler-age children by asking them to jump three times – if they couldn't, she knew they were really sick and not faking it. Kids under 5 are not likely to fake being sick unless it's learned behaviour (they can often suddenly say they have a sore back if you have one, for example, and will learn from you how to react to hurts and pains).

For books on recognising and dealing with illnesses see "More info & contacts" at the end of this book.

When to go to a hospital emergency department with a child

If you're very worried about your kid and you can't go to your local doctor because it's late at night or a weekend, you may need to go to the nearest hospital emergency (A&E) department. Please be aware, though, that casualty areas are only for emergencies, and that you may have to wait a long time in a crowded, brightly lit area and then see an overworked doctor or nurse. So if you are anxious about, but not freaked out by, your child's symptoms, a good alternative to waiting in casualty can be to call NHS Direct on 0845 4647. A nurse may be able to advise on the best steps to take. Or, ring your local GP's out-of-hours service requesting a home visit. Call and see how quickly the doctor can come: sick children will be a priority.

Looking after a sick child

- ★ Sick babies can be carried in a sling or wheeled about the house with you in a pram.
- ★ With a toddler, help the patient camp out in the room you're working in. Make up a bed on the sofa with toy friends and settle the patient in for the day so they're not isolated; or move an armchair into their bedroom with some reading, the phone or work you can do there. If vomiting or pooing is not a possibility, the parental bed can be a good haven.
- ★ Sick kids often sleep a lot as a natural defence or because of the sedative effect of medicines such as painkillers or cough suppressants. Don't use painkillers to sedate: it's not good for kids to have too many (see p. 9 for more detail).

★ Don't insist on games or activities – sometimes kids are too ill to do anything but lie about.

★ Read them a favourite book or two or play some sleepy-time or relaxing music.

★ Don't let them veg out for ages in front of the TV or new DVDs. The younger the child, the more it can addle their brain when they're sick – too many new concepts to take in. Tried and trusted, quieter programmes can be useful.

★ Offer simple food and healthy staples. Old-fashioned comfort food such as custard or mashed potatoes can be good, depending on the illness. Upset tummies usually mean a (temporarily) very restricted diet (we'll get to that), and kids with stuffed-up noses can't taste anything. Sore mouths and throats often mean food rejection.

★ Don't forget to change the sheets after an illness to freshen up, and get some outside air into the room during an illness if possible and definitely after.

★ You want to be as sympathetic as possible without making being ill a great adventure preferable to being up.

★ If you've had to cancel work or something else important to be at home, make sure you plot against the illness in partnership with your kid ("I can't wait to go to the park! Let's go as soon as you're better!") rather than resenting your child for being ill ("I hope you're better tomorrow because I missed some important things at work today").

★ Put your kid in a tepid bath if the weather is horribly hot, or a warm one can be relaxing if it's cold. If your child doesn't want one, try a flannel or "sponge" bath. The patient can try a dry wash of teddy first.

★ Reality check: you may have to re-establish your child's sleeping routine after an illness.

Giving medicines

Most children's medicines come as a liquid that can be sucked up into a dropper or syringe (without the needle bit, obviously) and squirted into the child's mouth; or it can be given on a spoon or in a tiny measuring cup. The dropper, spoon or measuring cup may come with the medicine or you can buy them separately at the chemist.

It's always handy to teach your kid how to take medicine from a dropper as soon as possible. Try to make it a game.

In cases of full-on, arched-back rebellion, when taking the medicine immediately is imperative, hold the child's nose so they have to open their mouth, squirt it in and then hold the mouth closed until it's swallowed. This is of course an absolutely last resort and can usually be avoided by reassurance or sneakiness.

If you have to disguise medicine in a mouthful of something, use a tiny amount of breast or formula milk for a baby or, say, a spoonful of food such as ice cream for older kids. It's no good putting medicine in a glass of juice because they'll only drink 56.78 percent of the juice and then you'll have no idea how much of it was medicine. Some children's medicines can be over-flavoured and are brightly coloured, which is guaranteed to make any baby or fussy toddler deeply suspicious.

Some parents have success with bribery – "You take your medicine, you get a sticker or a star on a chart."

PAINKILLERS: PARACETAMOL AND IBUPROFEN

★ Ask your doctor or pharmacist for advice on paracetamol and ibuprofen for babies over 3 months and kids, and keep a supply on hand. They come under different brand names. (Painkillers should be given to children under 3 months old only at the direction of your doctor.) Although entirely safe for most babies and toddlers, painkillers containing ibuprofen can cause side effects in individual kids, including some who have asthma. As well as dulling or removing pain, paracetamol is commonly used for bringing down a temperature, although both will do this (but see the section "Fever and high temperature" later in the chapter).

★ Paracetamol isn't designed to be used all day every day, for several days in a row, without medical supervision: a whacking great paracetamol overdose can cause permanent liver shutdown. Long-term use or longer-than-recommended doses of ibuprofen cause tummy upsets and bleeding. Both should be kept out of reach and locked away.

★ Don't ever exceed the dose – more will not kill pain quicker or more efficiently. The recommended dose should do it within 20 minutes. If it doesn't, you'll be needing medical advice.

★ If you do accidentally give too much medicine, don't panic. Ring NHS Direct immediately (0845 4647) and let them know how much you've given. Ibuprofen should not be given to kids with asthma as it's been known to make it worse.

★ Aspirin or soluble aspirin should not be given to kids under 16, as in rare cases it can contribute to Reye's syndrome, a liver failure and brain inflammation leading to convulsions and coma, with a high death rate (10 to 25 percent).

Never leave a bottle of medicine where kids can reach it, regardless of "child-proof" lids.

> *"Try putting your baby's medicine into an upturned teat and let them suck it like it was on a bottle."* SAMANTHA

> *"My kids will take medicine off the 'magic spoon' (we got it out of the kids' Nurofen packet)."* PRUE

Complementary therapies

Many people see an alternative practitioner – yours should understand when it's necessary to have a medical diagnosis before complementary treatments. Just treating symptoms might allow an underlying cause to go unnoticed. Complementary therapies are good for minor ailments when the cause is indisputable. Your practitioner should be both qualified and experienced in children's remedies, and the cause of the ailment should be fully medically established. Herbalists should be told about any medications the child is on, and doctors told of any herbal remedies the kid is taking as well. Sensible herbalists and naturopaths will not recommend their remedies alone for serious illnesses or injuries. So far, there have been no accepted scientific studies which show homeopathic remedies work better than a placebo, while some traditional, naturopathic or herbal remedies do have scientific backing. As with medical treatment, parents will have to make themselves aware of specific latest research.

Mindful of the long list of powerful and complicated aromatherapy essential oils, I should say that small children should probably only be given drops of eucalyptus oil on their hanky or pillow (to combat the sniffles) or a drop of lavender oil in their bath for relaxation. Essential oils should not be applied neat to the skin. Don't use aromatherapy candles or burners for children, and never leave these (or anything else with an unprotected flame) untended in a room a child is in.

When you get ill too

This is when you find out who your real friends and actually helpful relatives are. Many people want to stay away when there is illness in the home. It can be especially daunting, even frightening, when you are a sole parent and have been literally laid out by something really serious. Don't be afraid to ask friends and family for help, insisting if necessary.

Carer fatigue

I never used to understand what people meant when they said that having an ill child was difficult. Now I understand it can mean hours and hours of grinding exhaustion and sacrifice, the kind of worry that makes you realise you never really had a worry before, and the total inability to do anything at all apart from tend to the patient, get them to and from the doctor and wash mega kilos of sickie bed linen, jarmies and towels. Most children who are ill wake up a lot, distressed, and even if *they* go straight back to sleep *you* might lie awake until the next "alarm". If you have a partner, try to alternate the sleepless nights. One partner can wear earplugs or sleep in the furthest room when it's not their turn on shift.

If your child is in childcare or nursery, use the first few days they're well and back there to get some sleep during the day. Otherwise see if you can get help from a friend or relative so that you catch up on your sleep. The more tired (or the sicker) you are, the harder it is to have good judgement and stay patient.

The common illnesses and conditions that follow in the rest of this chapter are in no particular order except that they start with the more temporary and common ones and end with the more long-term conditions.

fever and High temperature

We are all so attuned to the idea that fevers are scary, it can be a horrible shock to pick up your baby or toddler and realise they're "burning up". It's comforting to know that most fevers are friends: they have a sensible purpose – it's the body's way of "burning off" germs. Your kid's immune system is doing its job. Almost all children recover quickly and without problems from a fever. In a very small number of children, the fever may not improve or they develop other symptoms, which can be a sign of serious illness or infection. If you are concerned about your child's fever, call your GP, or NHS Direct on 0845 4647.

One of the quickest ways to see if a baby has a fever is to put the back of your hand against their tummy (their forehead and extremities may have been in a cold wind or near a heater and are not as close to the body's core temperature). If it feels very hot, there's probably a fever.

A febrile convulsion

It's rare, but a rapid rise in temperature can cause a "febrile convulsion", or fit, which causes the eyes to roll back and the baby or kid to shake and jerk. A fit is scary but usually takes only a few minutes and has no lasting effects, and doesn't cause brain damage or death. (A tendency to have fits sometimes runs in the family.) Call an ambulance if you're freaked out (let's face it, who wouldn't be?) but it'll probably all be over before they get to your place, with no harm done except to your nerves.

Doctors say it's likely that the rapid rate of the temperature rise causes a fit rather than a magic high number such as forty degrees Celsius. So by the time you know your kid has a high temperature, if they haven't had a fit they're probably not going to. Remember: the vast majority of kids never have febrile convulsions and those who do are not harmed by them.

Ways to treat a fever

★ If your baby or child has a convulsion, call an ambulance on 999.

★ Don't keep the kid too bundled up, and don't use ice or anything else sudden to "bring down" a temperature.

★ If the kid is in pain or miserable, give them a dose of paracetamol, according to the instructions on the label. If they're jaunty, let the fever fight the illness.

★ See a doctor if your kid has other worrying symptoms, such as being "not themselves", cranky, listless, confused, off their food or having a rash, repeated vomiting or breathing changes. You'll probably want to take a baby under 6 months to the doctor if you feel they have a high temperature, to rule out anything worrying.

★ If you're frightened by the high temperature or it's 4am and you're feeling exhausted, you can use a dose of paracetamol to bring down the fever and see a doctor the next day.

The usual advice is that a baby under 6 months with a fever over 37.5 degrees should be seen as soon as possible by a GP. For a baby older than that, if the temperature is over 38.5 for more than four hours, or comes and goes at that high level, also see your doctor.

gastro (tummy bug)

"When they say they have a tummy ache and turn a shade of green they ARE going to vomit." **TRACEY**

We're talking here about an upset tummy – the vomiting and diarrhoea associated with a short-term bug rather than something longer term such as a tummy parasite, or the one-off vomiting caused by stress,

★ The baby or kid has repeated runny poos over the course of 24 hours.

★ Their skin feels dry and papery or cold and clammy and is paler than usual.

★ The skin on a baby's fontanelle (the small, soft part of the top of their head) looks sunken.

★ Foul breath.

★ A dry mouth, lips and tongue.

★ The face and eyes look sunken.

★ A spaced-out, glazed look.

★ There's less wee than usual or fewer wet nappies.

★ The wee is darker coloured than usual (this is sometimes hard to see if they're wearing a nappy).

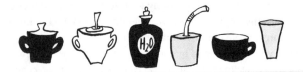

coughing or getting a chunk of apple caught in the throat. The throwing up is often very upsetting for a baby or kid, especially if it wakes them or they don't know what's happening.

Generally vomiting plus diarrhoea plus fever means you need to see your doctor, although it's almost certainly a short-term bout. The main danger, to babies in particular, is dehydration if they're too sick to keep down or keep drinking fluids. This can happen quite quickly to babies: 24 hours of vomiting and diarrhoea can be enough. If you can't rehydrate them, they need to go to hospital to be sedated and go on a nice drip of fluids and mineral salts for a day or so. Scary for you, but standard procedure.

Gastro is caused by a virus picked up anywhere really, but often in a place where there's a concentration of other kids; by bacteria, perhaps in contaminated food (food poisoning) or, in rare cases, by a rather violent allergic reaction. Symptoms are usually most full-on for the first 24 hours, and the diarrhoea often lasts longer than the vomiting. There may be only throwing up or only diarrhoea.

A viral case usually comes on suddenly: the kid complains of feeling nauseated or goes quiet, then suddenly vomits. It may be accompanied by other charming features such as runny poo and sniffly cold symptoms. This is the most common, catching kind.

A bacterial gastro such as food poisoning usually comes on within about 12 to 48 hours of contact. The food involved can be anything from a tiny bit of old milk not rinsed out of an otherwise clean formula bottle to something that touched a surface contaminated by raw chicken. Tummy cramps and explosive poo often come first, followed by vomiting. It normally lasts two to three days.

Treatment for gastro

There's not much in the way of medication you can give for gastro – usually you have to ride it out by doing the following:

★ Help your baby or child and be with them while they are vomiting, then clean up as soon as you can.

★ Give them reassurance and cuddles. Throwing up is an unpleasant experience and they need comforting and soothing.

★ Rest your child's tummy from rich foods (see "What not to feed a kid with gastro" further on). Do this for a day – more if it seems to be still upset.

★ Rehydration is the important issue. Give your kid lots of fluids. Basically keep offering the breast, bottle or cup as often as you can to babies. Keep a drink next to a child who is old enough to help themselves and also offer it to them often.

You can get a rehydration formula from the chemist (you may need a prescription, but some can be bought in bottles or sachets over the counter). It needs to be appropriate for your child's age and contain the right mineral salts as well as fluids. Some can even be frozen as "icy poles" to make them more attractive to kids. This is what you need, not flat lemonade. Remember that some chemists will home deliver.

★ Keep cross-infection to a minimum by washing all utensils, sick bowls, towels and jarmies in hot, soapy water.

★ Always take a child of any age to the doctor if you're worried or if there are any signs of dehydration such as no wet nappies or wee for ten hours; dry mouth, tongue or lips; weakness; fast or slow breathing; severe tiredness or coldness to the touch.

BABIES UNDER 3 MONTHS WITH GASTRO

★ After twelve hours of gastro head off to the doctor just to make sure it's all okay: ask for advice about rehydrating.

★ If your baby is breastfed, keep offering breast milk regularly.

★ If they're a formula-fed baby, ask your doctor whether you should try a special rehydration formula for their age from the pharmacy in their bottle for a day, then their own formula at half-strength for a day, before going back to normal. Some babies come good suddenly and can probably go straight back onto their formula.

OLDER BABIES (3 MONTHS TO 1 YEAR) WITH GASTRO

★ See your doctor if the vomiting and diarrhoea last longer than 48 hours or call NHS Direct (0845 4647) if concerned.

★ Your baby should go back on breast or formula milk as soon as possible.

TODDLERS (OVER 1 YEAR) WITH GASTRO

★ Keep giving plain water and clear fruit juice diluted 1:1 with water or rehydration fluids or "icy poles" from the chemist.

★ Never assume a toddler knows what's going on. Explain why you're offering different foods and drinks, why you're going to the doctor, why it's good to stay quietly at home.

★ A kid old enough to understand (but who may have forgotten what throwing up is) should be reassured that the situation will end soon, that they have a germ that is making their tummy have a tantrum and that you're trying to fix it as fast as you can but sometimes it may take until tomorrow (anything longer is virtually incomprehensible).

★ If a toddler or a child with gastro wants to eat, feed them bland things and don't worry too much – they will be getting a few nutrients even if they throw up everything soon after (see "What to feed a kid with gastro", which follows).

★ The NHS recommend that you see your doctor if the vomiting and diarrhoea last longer than five days, but call NHS Direct (0845 4647) sooner if you are worried.

WHAT TO FEED A KID WITH GASTRO

Don't force feed – start food when your child is ready. Try:

★ plain cooked rice and pasta
★ rice pudding
★ fingers of dry toast or bread
★ plain dry biscuits, with reduced salt
★ porridge made with water
★ mashed potatoes
★ puréed, mashed or sieved frozen blueberries and raspberries or little bits of fresh fruit
★ plain soya milk
★ grated or paper-thin apple slices
★ stewed pear

17

- ⭐ banana
- ⭐ mashed carrot or courgettes
- ⭐ jelly
- ⭐ finely chopped steamed chicken breast
- ⭐ plain home-made chicken soup

WHAT NOT TO FEED A KID WITH GASTRO

- ⭐ Only plain water for longer than 24 hours: the body needs more nutrients than that.

PRACTICAL TIPS FOR LIVING WITH THE VOMITS

Sick bowl

Protect yourself and bedding from sudden vomits by teaching your child as soon as possible to use a sick bowl. Make sure you have a couple of non-metal sick bowls or buckets (who wants to see their reflection at that point?) and plenty of layers of towels to avoid getting vomit on the bed or furniture. The towels will have to be washed in very hot water and an antibacterial washing powder such as a nappy one. The bowl the child uses will have to be disinfected with boiling water at intervals too, with the spare kept in circulation in case there's a need while the other one's being washed.

Stripping the bed

When a kid throws up in bed, it's all hands on deck. This is why you never throw out old, threadbare towels – keep all the towels you can.

Soothe the kid thoroughly first, then completely clean them with a nice warm flannel and a soap substitute, paying special attention to face, hands and hair. Rinse off the soap substitute, wrap your darling in a clean towel and prop them in a corner or on a beanbag where they can't fall over (but never leave a baby on a beanbag while you go into another room). Explain that the vomiting might happen again but it might not, and what's causing it. Dress them in loose clothes

- ★ Full-strength fruit juice or full-strength lemonade because both are too sugary and can stimulate diarrhoea – water it down to at least 1:1.
- ★ Flat lemonade or sugar dissolved in water – it's much better to get a rehydration formula from the chemist.
- ★ Bottled electrolyte and sports drinks: they're for adults.
- ★ Spicy, acidic or rich foods, chocolate, junk foods, sweets, cake and other sugary things: these can make the diarrhoea worse.
- ★ Salty things: these can increase dehydration.

you'll be able to get off easily if they're sick again. Don't assume they won't vomit again or that there's "nothing left to come up": protect the immediate area.

Strip the bed of all the sheets and any bedding with vomit on it and soak up any extra vomit with old or used towels. Clean any vomit-touched surfaces with antibacterial spray (or similar) and another towel. Explain that you're putting all the bedding, jarmies, towels and vomity stuffed-animals in the washing machine, or leave everything in a pile to take away later.

Come back; have a cuddle and remake the bed: if you don't have a waterproof mattress protector use a couple of layers of old towels. Make up a top sheet with a bath towel that folds back to protect the top layer of sheet, duvet or bedspread. Have the sick bowl ready next to the bed before the child gets back in. Prop up an older child with pillows and make sure the only toys that stay are washable. (We've had to have Pinky re-upholstered twice and it's quite undignified.) Offer them a drink of water. Reassuringly tuck them in and send them off to sleep if possible.

Before loading the washing machine rinse off anything chunky, do a short but adequately cleansing washing-machine load with antibacterial powder in hot water.

If you're unlucky, do it all again. Of course if there are two adults divvying up the actions just described it will work even better.

- ★ Anti-diarrhoea medicines unless your doctor prescribed them specifically for this bout of illness (these medicines are rarely given and hardly ever to babies).
- ★ Milk and other dairy food because they're too fatty.

SNiffLes aNd CoLds

Home remedies

- ★ A steam vaporiser can be bought from a pharmacy. You fill them with water and they keep pushing steam into the child's room at night – this helps keep the airways open and greatly reduces a stuffed nose and coughing. Some people put eucalyptus drops in, but that's not necessary for them to work effectively.
- ★ A vapour rub (from the chemist) on the chest for toddlers may help clear the schnozz.
- ★ Add one drop of eucalyptus oil to the bath.
- ★ Eucalyptus drops on the pillow, underneath the pillow case, might help too.
- ★ Elevate the head of the bed with a few volumes of the *Yellow Pages* – the mucus will drain down.
- ★ Books or music can be soothing.

Coughs

- ★ A wheezy cough: this could indicate asthma and should always be checked by a doctor.
- ★ A cough that ends in a heaving or barking sound (a "whoop") as the baby or child tries to take in air: this should also always be checked by a doctor.
- ★ A croupy cough (one with lots of rattly phlegm in the chest): this can often be suddenly improved by placing a steam vaporiser in the bedroom at night.

Pharmacy shelves are chockers with expensive cold, cough and sniffle remedies for kids but doctors are dubious about their effect on illness. A honey and lemon drink could well be just as good. Remember that children's cough medicines must be literally made for children – never use a smaller dose of an adult cough mixture – and that most have quite a strong sedative as well as a cough suppressant in them. So generally they are most helpful at night to let a kid get some sleep (and you too) if that's what's become necessary.

Babies under 1 year mustn't have off-the-shelf decongestant cough mixtures: these must be prescribed for them by a doctor.

> *"Mums tend to see changes in a condition where dads see variations from the normal state. Listen and act on both concerns."* **GRAHAM**

ear problems

Lots of babies and small kids get ear trouble, usually after a cold or other virus. Although unusual in a tiny baby under a couple of months old, after that it can be a battle, with some kids having constant problems for years. Most kids will have at least one ear infection before school starts. The three main types of ear condition are given below. (If you want to have your child's hearing tested call your GP's surgery.)

Outer ear infection

This is often caused by "picking something up at the pool". You can see the ear is red, with maybe a discharge – older kids may say it feels

EARS

* See a doctor if there is ear pain, redness, pulling at an ear associated with pain (not the typical baby "What's this thing on my head I've just discovered?" behaviour), perceived or suspected hearing trouble, or a discharge from the ear.

* If you need to give ear drops, have your child lie down with their head sideways on your lap and let gravity help you. Say it won't hurt (if that's true) but might feel wet or tickly while the drops are draining into the ear.

* Don't push anything, even a cotton bud, into a baby's or a kid's ear. Clean the bit you can reach with a flannel.

blocked or sore. It may go away by itself but should be seen by your GP and may need antibiotics or steroid medicines.

Middle ear infection

Inside everyone's ear is a thing called a eustachian tube that drains any fluid from the middle ear, which is protected from the outside world by the eardrum. In kids under about 3 the tube is often rather horizontal before developing a downward angle so fluid can drain away. If the fluid doesn't drain and sits there, it can get very infected and yucky and can eventually burst out of the eardrum, causing sudden pain (or it can cause "glue" ear – more on that coming up).

The symptoms are usually bad earache and a lack of interest in food (because it hurts to swallow). Unfortunately a little baby or toddler may not be able to understand and articulate the pain or show you where it is. The early signs may be listlessness, tears and deafness that might be obvious or not.

The first treatment is pain relief – usually the label dosage of paracetamol for the correct age. If the yuck has burst through the eardrum, the pain of the pressure will be released and the drum will probably heal nicely by itself (not that you'd want this to happen repeatedly). Antibiotics can be used to clear up the infection behind the ear, but the problem is likely to recur until (or if) the tube starts draining properly.

"Glue" ear

The ear becomes blocked when fluid can't drain away or doesn't burst through the eardrum, but it's not necessarily infected. There's no pain, but there is significant, partial to total hearing loss. Quite often someone else notices it first – a childcare worker or a relative. Kids can get very good at lip reading and finding other ways around their deafness. Parents often first realise when a child has their back to them and doesn't respond to questions, or keeps asking for the music or TV to be turned up.

In persistent cases or where the alternative is a partial or complete deafness in one or both ears that would lead to learning and social difficulties, the kid may have to have an operation under general anaesthetic to insert "grommets". These are little eyelets holding open holes in the eardrum so that the fluid can drain out. Kids can swim with grommets in, but not dive or jump in the pool or ocean waves in case water pounds into their inner ear. After a few months grommets drop out of the ear naturally and the drum heals itself.

Incidentally those ear candle things (under various brand names) that some people burn outside a kid's ear, which are supposed to draw out a blockage, are completely useless. Even if a candle could draw material towards it, there's an eardrum in the way, making it impossible. And lighted candles should be kept away from children's heads! "Natural" remedy ear drops should only be used when your doctor is certain the eardrum has not been perforated.

PART 2
immunisation

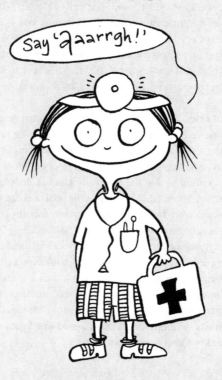

Part 2: immunisation

Why we need to immunise

Do you need to worry about the old-fashioned diseases that seem to have disappeared? Well, yes, if your child hasn't been immunised, because sadly, some of these "old-fashioned" diseases haven't actually disappeared at all. They lurk about quietly in the background and try to make a comeback every now and again – sometimes with deadly results.

The only way to worry a lot less about their health is to have your children fully immunised – given all the vaccines recommended by the NHS schedule (listed soon). That way you know you've protected them as much as you can, and when they get sick, it's not likely to be something really scary.

Luckily for us, we have this free and efficient immunisation programme for our kids which has tackled the spread of dangerous childhood diseases. These vaccines used in the immunisation programme were invented by doctors and scientists desperate to save children from the devastating effects of childhood diseases. Now they're available from your nearest health centre or doctor's surgery.

Because of the immunisation programme, most UK kids are now protected by a "herd immunity" – meaning that when enough children are immunised, the spread of disease is held at bay. The problem comes when those levels of immunisation begin to fall; individual kids are left unprotected and the "old" diseases take the opportunity to start spreading again.

This has just happened in the UK. In April 2009 the Health Protection Agency reported an "unprecedented" rise in measles cases. Measles can kill, and does kill tens of thousands of kids elsewhere, each year. (This is recently down from hundreds of thousands a year, due to immunisation programmes worldwide.)

What we're protecting kids from

In the developing world, where these diseases are more prevalent, parents will sometimes queue for days in a desperate effort to get their babies and kids protected. Unlike most of us nowadays, they've seen what happens when these diseases take hold.

Immunisations now also protect British children against tetanus, which is always around in dirt, and can cause nerve-system paralysis and death. Along with diphtheria, which causes a swelling in the throat, tetanus is still a big killer of children overseas. So is measles.

Despite polio still being present only a plane ride away in some developing countries, the UK has been almost free of polio since mass immunisation of children began in the 1950s. Before that, polio epidemics struck repeatedly, causing widespread panic, and many children's legs were permanently paralysed. Before the vaccine was introduced for pertussis (whooping cough), up to 120,000 babies and children caught the disease each year, and many died. Also on the schedule hit-list are mumps and rubella (German measles).

More recently, vaccines have been developed so that British kids are protected against dangerous lung diseases such as *Haemophilus influenzae* type b (Hib for short) and pneumococcal infection. Both of these serious illnesses can lead to meningitis. A chicken pox vaccine is now available, but is not routine.

Other, "non-routine" vaccinations are also a good idea if you're travelling to certain areas. Typhoid, cholera and yellow fever are the sort of "extras" you'll need to consider when travelling to some countries.

Unfortunately for parents who don't have medical degrees, it can be nigh on impossible to know whether a fever or sudden bout of "floppy" disinterest is just a miserable common bug with no long-term effects, or something far more worrying, such as measles, mumps or meningitis, or even one of the new strains of flu associated with birds, pigs or whatever's next. Part 3 of this booklet, Childhood diseases & what to do about them, will help you identify symptoms of serious diseases, tell you the likely treatments, and explain why immunisation is a good idea to prevent them, in each case.

CURRENT ROUTINE CHILDHOOD IMMUNISATION SCHEDULE

Although the list of vaccines at each scheduled age looks daunting, a few vaccines can be combined in the same injection so there probably won't be more than two jabs at any appointment, except at four months when there'll be three. The following schedule of free vaccines operated at July 2009:

* **two months** – first dose for diphtheria, tetanus, pertussis, polio, Hib, pneumococcal infection.
* **three months** – second dose for diphtheria, tetanus, pertussis, polio, Hib; first dose for meningitis C.
* **four months** – third dose for diphtheria, tetanus, pertussis, polio, Hib; second dose for pneumococcal infection and meningitis C.
* **around twelve months** – boosters for Hib and meningitis C.
* **around thirteen months** – first dose for measles, mumps, rubella; booster for pneumococcal infection.
* **three years four months to five years old** – fourth dose of diphtheria, tetanus, pertussis, polio, and second dose for measles, mumps, rubella.

The next scheduled jabs are adolescent boosters for diphtheria, tetanus and polio and, for girls, the HPV (human papillomavirus) jabs, which protect against cervical cancer.

Children considered "at risk" may be targeted for extra, free vaccines such as BCG (to protect against tuberculosis) or hepatitis B: ask your GP if you are eligible.

Teddy's had 27 injections

Vaccines that may be required for travel may have to be paid for.

How does a vaccine work?

Vaccines against bacterial disease usually contain a form of the bacteria or toxin that causes the disease it will protect against. A tiny bit of, let's say, Hib bacteria has been treated so it can't actually cause the disease itself but prompts the body to produce antibodies – protection against the disease. In some cases an inactive component of the bacteria (for example, its sugar coating) is mixed with a protein known to help it produce the required reaction in a young body.

A vaccine might also contain a preservative and barely detectable traces of formaldehyde, used to kill the contagious bit of the bacteria or virus in the lab. Some vaccines that protect against viruses are "live" but have been altered so that they are a very weak form of the virus. They produce immunity but don't cause the disease. Initially a vaccine is tested on laboratory animals, then larger animals, then finally on human volunteers. Results are reported, published and checked by government licensors.

getting an immunisation

If you have a lot of questions you'd like answered, it's probably best to go to your practice nurse, doctor or health visitor. They should ask you some questions to make sure the vaccine is right for your child and your family, and that there are no previous illnesses or allergic conditions that mean your child should see an immunisation specialist at your local hospital.

If your kid is quite sick and has a fever, it's probably best to postpone the immunisation in case it's harder to spot any side effects of the vaccination. If your kid has sneezes, sniffles or an ordinary old cold it's almost always fine to go ahead with the immunisation, but ask if you're worried.

How to help a child on injection day

Babies usually just look momentarily horrified and accusing when they get their injections, and cry briefly until they're cuddled and distracted, perhaps by a breastfeed or bottlefeed. Older kids usually are stoical or cry a little and they too forget the pain moments later, especially when cunningly distracted. You may be surprised to see how slender and quick the disposable needle is these days.

Have tissues on-hand for tears, two special treats for an older baby or small child, a comforting toy or other item. The following things should help with toddlers and nursery-age children:

★ There is usually no point in describing the scene to a kid or building up anticipation (which is likely to be fearful) – but be guided by your specialist knowledge of your child. Jennifer Irwin, an immunisation nurse, says "Think about how much preparation your child needs before any new experience. Sometimes it is good to have a story or two a day or so before or perhaps some play with a toy medical

29

kit to prepare." You can ask your playgroup or childcare centre to have a group chat about it.

★ Don't give a toddler the option of saying "no" to a jab. This is one of the times as a parent you need to gently tell them what's going to happen, not ask them if it's okay with them, or wait until they think it's a good idea to have a jab.

★ At the actual time be matter of fact about having an injection; don't build it up to be important or scary.

★ Never say "Don't cry."

★ Explain (even if it's been explained before) that the nurse or doctor is going to put some very special medicine inside them to stop them from getting bad illnesses, and that the nurse or doctor is going to use a needle and it will only take a second.

★ If asked, don't pretend that it won't hurt. Say it might sting for a short time but you'll have a special surprise treat ready for them straight afterwards.

★ You will be asked to hold the kid firmly to help them be very still. Try to make this feel cuddly rather than restraining.

★ Distraction is the key. Most kids prefer to look away, but some like to watch: either is fine. Some like a cartoon adhesive strip over the injection spot.

★ Immediately afterwards ask the kid to make a choice between, say, a sticker or a jelly bean: a choice of treats is very distracting and will usually stop any crying.

★ Praise them for sitting still during the injection and having it. Make a fuss of them.

★ You can press on the injection site afterwards to dull the stinging, but don't massage it.

★ If the injection site is red and sore afterwards, a cool pack can be held gently on it and a usual dose of baby or child paracetamol (see label) could be given.

★ Children will appreciate a "debriefing" so have a chat about why they had the injection and how they're protected against special illnesses now. Keep up the praise.

★ The site of the injection may be sore to the touch for a few days. This is because injection into soft tissues can cause low-level bruising.

★ Ask your doctor or nurse for any side effects you should keep an eye out for and what to do if they appear.

Reactions

A dose of infant paracetamol or ibuprofen liquid can help reduce your child's fever (see the box on painkillers on p. 9). You may need to give a second dose four to six hours later. Most children show no reaction at all, apart from being a bit affronted and up for a major bribe straight after the injection. Breast or bottle milk or drinks can also be comforting. If there is a fever call NHS Direct on 0845 4647; it might not be the immunisation that is causing the high temperature. (Young children pick up new infections often but usually fight them off.) You can give paracetamol to bring a fever down, but only if your kid is in pain or miserable. A sudden high fever can cause a brief fit. Fever does not cause brain damage. If there is a convulsion, call an ambulance on 999 immediately: it's best to be safe.

In extremely exceptional cases, vaccination can cause anaphylactic shock, an immediate allergic reaction. Because babies and small children rarely faint after an injection, a loss of consciousness should be treated as anaphylaxis – a life-threatening emergency because it can cause throat swelling leading to suffocation. If it's going to happen, it will almost certainly do so within five minutes of the injection. Treatment is usually a swift adrenaline injection, possibly extra oxygen and always a trip to hospital for observation. (A nurse giving one hundred immunisations a week for 52 weeks a year would see one of these reactions once every two hundred years. And she'd be very wrinkly by then too.)

If your child has had a reaction to an injection, such as a high fever, talk about it with your doctor or health visitor, or call NHS direct on 0845 4647.

for and against

There are some very heated debates about vaccinations. At the extremes there are doctors who say it isn't worth discussing the fact that a relatively tiny number of kids are damaged by vaccines because it's far fewer than those who would have died from the diseases if there had been no vaccinations; and at the other end there are some nutty anti-vaccinators who say extremely dodgy stuff, often on their websites, including this: "Children who were breastfed and are well looked after have an immune system which will protect them against all diseases." (This, frankly, is a big fat fib.)

Parents don't always look at the big picture and I think doctors need to understand this. We are usually more worried about what effect a vaccine might have on our individual tiny person than thrilled to participate in a disease-eradication public health programme. When doctors say there's only a one-in-a-million chance of a serious vaccination reaction such as a seizure, they should remember we're all worried that our baby might be that one in a million. (For the vast majority of parents, it gets easier by the second lot of scheduled jabs because the first ones caused no problems at all.)

parents in the middle

Parents with legitimate questions can be treated like rabid twits by

All immunisations administered to children are logged in the Personal Child Health Record (the "red book"), which is issued at birth for all babies and kept by the parents. Nurseries and schools in the UK do not usually require proof of immunisation, but you may be required to show some record when entering another country.

both sides. On the one hand the "information" given to them in anti-vaccination books and on websites is most often a shocking mix of lies, twisted statistics and accusations totally irrelevant to UK vaccines. On the other hand a few worried parents say they have been bullied by doctors instead of being given information respectfully. (Time to find another GP if you feel that's the case: the majority will talk to you sensibly about concerns.)

Most people have already made up their mind about what they think of vaccines by the time they have children. Some get whatever's on the schedule, no questions asked. A few vehemently oppose vaccinations and won't be swayed by any facts presented. The following is really for people who want more info before closing their eyes, crossing their fingers and jumping (a time-honoured, metaphorical parent-decision-making technique).

Despite the claims of many anti-vaccine lobbyists, the dedicated medical staff who immunise children are, hey, *probably not* part of some bizarre, worldwide, shifty-eyed conspiracy to make money for drug companies, and *probably not* brainwashed, robotic devotees of weird science. And it seems equally evident that sadly a very, very small number of individual children among millions may be harmed by a vaccine. In a perfect world each child's reactions would be perfectly predictable, each child with a medical predisposition would have obvious symptoms, and each vaccine dose would be individually tailored to the levels of immunity in each child without needing blood to be taken with yet another injection. Ultimately parents will have to weigh up the tiny statistical risk for their child against the protection from dangerous diseases.

arguments about immunisation

Additives

Some anti-vaccination activists have said that mercury in childhood vaccines was causing health problems. As there is no mercury (thiomersal) used in any of the UK injections on the routine schedule for kids there's no point in arguing the issue here, although the idea has been discredited. Despite claims of most anti-vaccination books and websites, you can be assured that all routine childhood vaccines are free of mercury. If you're worried, ask your doctor to get out the list of ingredients from the packet and take you through them.

There is a tiny amount of gelatin in one brand of MMR vaccine. But, the Muslim Council of Britain advises Muslims they are "duty-bound" to use life-saving preventative measures and the World Health Organization (WHO) website carries a statement endorsed by many Islamic medical scholars saying that the transformed gelatin can be considered "pure" and "permissible" to consume.

Vaccines do not cause autism

For a while there was a lot of publicity about whether the MMR (measles mumps rubella) vaccine caused autism. Now we know it doesn't.

It was a disagreement between all of the medical doctors in the world except for a tiny, tiny handful, versus some parents of sick children who suspected some damage was caused by the MMR vaccine. Some parents were concerned about giving three vaccines in one jab, preferring three injections spaced over time. This is because they believed that the immune system is too challenged by a multiple vaccine: another theory that doctors say has no supporting evidence and is disproven by the vast number of successful "triple" jabs.

In the late 1990s a UK digestion doctor called Andrew Wakefield worried parents by saying the MMR vaccine was linked to, or may cause, autism. His claims have now been totally disproved by every other study done previously or since on MMR and autism rates, and all reputable immune system and infectious diseases specialists. So now we know that MMR does not cause autism, nor do other vaccines.

Dr Nigel Curtis (Head of the Paediatric Infectious Diseases Unit at the Royal Children's Hospital Melbourne) says he understands why parents might blame an illness or condition on immunisation when it is not actually the culprit. Like other doctors, he points out that most kids who get autism do have the MMR injection – and most kids who don't have autism have it too.

"In any given day there are hundreds of babies having their MMR jab or preschoolers having the booster. That means any cold, cough, fever or dribble could be mistakenly blamed on the MMR even though it is probably not associated at all." If a child has a fit just before his injection, it's obviously caused by something else. If it happens five minutes after, it would have been blamed on the injection. Dr Curtis notes there is no connection between MMR and autism except that parents usually first notice signs of autism around the same age as the MMR injection is given. Research into the genetic causes of autism is continuing.

> *"The oldest inhabitants recollected no period at all at which measles had been so prevalent, or so fatal to infant existence; and many were the mournful [funeral] processions . . ."* **CHARLES DICKENS, *OLIVER TWIST*, 1837**

Common reasons for opposing immunisation

It isn't natural If you look at it that way, neither are tampons, anaesthetics, aeroplanes, men without beards, or HobNob biscuits. But they can all be quite useful on occasion.

The diseases don't exist any more Yes they do. Whooping cough cases are in many hospitals at any given time; measles cases have risen in England and Wales by 36 percent in the last year to well over 1000, nearly half of which are in London. Measles is so contagious that you can just walk past someone (with measles) in the street and come down with it.

Vaccines don't work Vaccines have been remarkably successful in reducing or eradicating diseases, but a very few vaccinated people can still contract a less virulent form of some of the diseases such as whooping cough. The medical establishment has always acknowledged this.

It is too much of a challenge to the child's immune system to give so many vaccinations, especially triple whammies Millions of children have taken the vaccine "load" without incident or injury. Some doctors say kids could take thousands of vaccines without a problem, and that's not provable either because it's a stupid and unnecessary suggestion. Doctors should just admit that they're offering a vast improvement on the past, when your child ran a much, much higher risk of pain, suffering, damage and death from preventable and rampant childhood diseases.

There are alternatives, such as breastfeeding and organic

food Several anti-vaccination lobbyists claim that you can protect your child from childhood diseases by breastfeeding and giving your child love, fresh air and organic food. This is a cruel and stupid lie that encourages some parents to think their dangerously sick or dying child wasn't given enough love, fresh air, unsightly carrots or breast milk when it has nothing to do with any of that. Some of the vaccine-preventable diseases are so wildly catching that an infected person walking into a room full of unimmunised people is likely to infect 90 percent of them, regardless of whether they were or are breastfed or how healthy they are. It is true that all those things will help build a better immune system. But that won't stop you from getting a very infectious disease.

There are homeopathic and herbal "alternatives" to vaccination These have been discredited by responsible herbalists and the British Homeopathy Association itself which says "There is no evidence to show that homeopathic medicines can be used instead of vaccination. The Faculty of Homeopathy recommends that immunisation is carried out in the usual way, unless there are strong medical contraindications."

Religious reasons Many people who oppose vaccination do so from a religious point of view: some Christians because of their idiosyncratic interpretation of the Bible.

Childhood diseases are mostly trivial, just requiring a couple of days in bed Oh, poop (see Part 3 on Childhood diseases & what to do about them). The World Health Organization (WHO) reports irregular outbreaks of all these diseases, including polio, whooping cough and diphtheria. Measles still kills hundreds of thousands of kids worldwide. It is certainly not true that childhood diseases are trivial for everyone, especially among children who are already at risk if their immune system is suppressed because they are undergoing treatment for a serious condition such as a transplant or cancer, or because they're babies in developing countries.

Pro-vaccination contacts

Your health visitor and GP will have all the official info on your immunisation schedule and can provide leaflets and info about individual vaccines and the diseases they protect against.

Most pro-vaccination books are heavy-going medical bricks that are only understandable to people in cardigans covered by white coats who use words such as "histocompatibility antigen specificities" in their lunch hour, and the books concentrate on the wider issue of public health rather than helping you to make an individual decision (for the more accessible books see "More info & contacts" at the end of this book).

Anti-vaccination contacts

I tried to find an anti-vaccination book or website that seems perfectly sober and reasonable. God knows I tried. But to be brutally candid, I only found nutty ones. This is one of the reasons why the writings are almost always self-published – big publishing houses and magazines won't touch them. Most of the authors fervently claimed that immunisation doesn't prevent disease – which is demonstrably not true. Almost all books, websites and articles in "alternative" magazines quote the same handful of self-described "researchers" or "experts".

You should be aware that many anti-vaccination websites and books repeat (as facts) claims that have been disproved – such as that vaccines cause autism, sudden infant death syndrome or cancer and that germs do not cause disease – or are unprovable. Most give lots of statistics, often obviously quoting from each other rather than primary sources, but on further investigation the statistics are selectively used or plain wrongly interpreted. Their info is almost always irrelevant to the UK (it's worth repeating that there's no mercury, known as thiomersal in routine UK child vaccines). They have said immunisation causes (variously) shaken baby syndrome, asthma, attention deficit disorder – in fact anything that has statistically risen since the introduction of vaccination including, to single out one US anti-vaccine activist, criminal behaviour (there is a whole book on the theory).

PART 3

CHILDHOOD DISEASES & WHAT TO DO ABOUT THEM

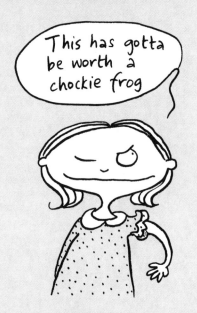

This has gotta be worth a chockie frog

PART 3: CHILDHOOD Diseases & WHAT TO DO ABOUT THEM

For each of the childhood diseases listed below, you will find symptoms, treatments and why a vaccine is necessary.

Chicken pox

SYMPTOMS AND EFFECTS

Chicken pox usually starts with a fever, listlessness, loss of appetite and a rash, followed by the tell tale spots, usually ten days to three weeks after catching the virus. The spots keep appearing for a few days and they all go through a process of becoming blistered, then itchy, before finally drying up. Scratching them may cause a scar. It is very contagious until the last sore has dried up.

HOW IT CAN BE SPREAD

Usually sneaky virus droplets – damp kid contact (infected clothes and bedding), sneezes etc. Chicken pox is most contagious one to two days before a rash appears. Early spots can be hard to detect and the disease remains contagious when the spots erupt.

TREATMENT

At home, you can wait out the week or go with painkillers and lots of fluids. Antibiotics won't help you get rid of the virus, but see your doctor in case complications are developing. A few advances have been made in chicken pox treatment. Nothing "cures" it – it has to run its course – but a special bath oil (ask your pharmacist) will help cut down the irritation of the itchy sores. Many UK doctors still recommend traditional calamine lotion, though there is a cooling, less drying gel also available at pharmacies. Ask your pharmacist about antihistamines (sometimes used for hayfever).

POSSIBLE SIDE EFFECTS OF THE VACCINE

Usual sore arm. Fever and rash are both common.

WHY WE NEED THE VACCINE

Chicken pox is not usually life threatening, but it is very miserable and irritating for most kids – some get nasty sores inside their mouths, down their throat, and on their genitals. While there is a vaccination against it, this is not part of the free UK childhood immunisation programme. (It may occasionally be offered to high-risk patients or to siblings of very sick children.) You will

have to ask for and pay for a chicken pox immunisation if you want one.
ALTERNATIVE TO THE VACCINE THAT WOULD GUARANTEE SAFETY
FROM INFECTION None.

Diphtheria

SYMPTOMS AND EFFECTS
Sore throat, fever, hoarse voice and cough. In severe cases a swelling causes
a blockage in the throat and can lead to suffocation, rarely paralysis, death in
up to ten percent of cases.
HOW IT CAN BE SPREAD
Sneezes, coughs, contact with bacteria on hand or tissue.
TREATMENT
Antibiotics and in some cases diphtheria antitoxin.
POSSIBLE SIDE EFFECTS OF THE VACCINE
See "Pertussis" (p. 46). (It's usually given together with pertussis and tetanus.)
WHY WE NEED THE VACCINE
One of the most deadly infectious diseases at the start of the 20th century.
Now virtually eradicated in many Western countries. (The former Soviet Union
still has outbreaks: one in the 1990s, when immunisation rates had fallen,
saw more than 150,000 cases and 5000 deaths.) Having the disease may
not necessarily protect against further infection. This is why you need five
injections: three as an infant, one as a toddler and one when 13–18 years old.
ALTERNATIVE TO THE VACCINE THAT WOULD GUARANTEE SAFETY
FROM INFECTION None.

Haemophilus influenzae type b (Hib)

SYMPTOMS AND EFFECTS
Not actually anything to do with flu virus but a bacteria. Can cause meningitis
(inflammation of brain lining, see p. 44) and septicaemia (blood poisoning),
hearing loss, brain damage, swelling in the throat that can suffocate, pneumo-
nia, joint and tissue infection, and death. A severe problem for the under-5s.
Most children who get it become very ill and need hospital treatment.
HOW IT CAN BE SPREAD
Coughs, sneezes and close contact.
TREATMENT
Emergency treatment with antibiotics.
POSSIBLE SIDE EFFECTS OF THE VACCINE
Low-grade fever, sore injection site (the thigh in babies up to age 1, and the
arm for older kids because the muscle is bigger then), nausea, joint pain.

Before Hib vaccine was introduced in 1992, around one in six hundred children developed some form of Hib disease by their fifth birthday, resulting in about thirty deaths every year and leaving about eighty children with deafness and permanent brain damage. Since the vaccine, cases of the disease in young children has fallen by 99 percent.

ALTERNATIVE TO THE VACCINE THAT WOULD GUARANTEE SAFETY FROM INFECTION None.

Measles

SYMPTOMS AND EFFECTS

Fever, cough, conjunctivitis, feeling miserable, irritability, exhaustion. Most common "target" is children aged 1–4; symptoms start off like a cold with a runny nose. In three to seven days, tiny red spots with white-blue centres can appear on the inside of your child's cheeks (but who knew?), then after three days to a week, a red rash of very tiny spots usually starts on the face and neck and spreads to the rest of the body. (Bear in mind it can be very difficult, if not impossible, to see a measles rash on dark skin.) Symptoms last about two weeks. After contact, it usually takes ten to fourteen days to show symptoms. Most kids will recover from measles, but rare complications can be very serious, including hepatitis and pneumonia. Measles can kill.

HOW IT CAN BE SPREAD

Sneezes, coughs or other contact. Astonishingly contagious virus, active for four days before and after the first appearance of the rash. There were 1445 new cases in the UK in 2008.

TREATMENT

Your doctor can do a simple saliva test to check for measles. If your child has it, stay in close contact with your doctor and inform everyone who has been around your child to get checked. There is no "treatment" that cures measles – you wait it out. For serious cases, hospitals may use anti-viral drugs. Paracetamol will bring fever down, and make sure they drink lots of water.

POSSIBLE SIDE EFFECTS OF THE VACCINE

Sore arm and in ten percent of children a mild fever and non-catchy rash, six to eleven days after the injection. Up to one in a million children may experience a seizure. A case of measles itself is much more likely to cause a seizure.

WHY WE NEED THE VACCINE

Measles used to be a common childhood disease in the UK. Between 1970 and 1988 there were between 50,000 and 1,000,000 cases and an average of thirteen deaths every year.

ALTERNATIVE TO THE VACCINE THAT WOULD GUARANTEE SAFETY
FROM INFECTION None. The MMR (measles mumps rubella) vaccine given
within 72 hours of contact, or an immunoglobulin injection given within
seven days, may or may not prevent or modify the disease.

Meningitis/Meningococcal disease

SYMPTOMS AND EFFECTS

Meningococcal disease can cause meningitis (which means brain lining swelling) and blood poisoning. The disease is very scary because the symptoms
– inflammation of the brain lining and spinal cord – can develop very suddenly within a couple of hours. In about one in ten cases it is not recognised
early enough and causes death. It is most dangerous in children under 5.
Meningitis is usually caused by the meningococcal bacteria, or another bacteria, or a virus. (See p. 51 for 24- hour phone lines with help on how to
recognise symptoms.)

Early warning signs of either meningitis can include severe pain in the legs
or hands, having very cold hands and feet, pale skin and blue-looking lips,
vomiting, fever, tiredness and headache.

Symptoms of bacterial meningitis can include a stiff neck and body or
appearing "floppy", rapid breathing, often with fever, pale and/or blotchy
skin and a very red or purple skin rash, not liking to be held, refusing to feed
and showing unusual levels of tiredness and unwillingness to wake up, crying
in an unusual way or moaning. Some small babies also have a slight swelling
of the soft, top part of their head. Bacterial meningitis can cause septicaemia
(pronounced sep-tee-seem-ia), a form of very fast-developing blood poisoning
which usually produces the distinctive red/purple rash of individual spots or
patches as well as the other usual viral meningitis symptoms (see below).This
blood poisoning can lead to amputations of affected limbs or death.

Symptoms of viral meningitis can include similar symptoms to those above
of bacterial meningitis, flu-like fevers with high and rising temperatures, aching
and headaches, nausea and vomiting, abnormal sensitivity to light. It usually
does not cause a distinctive rash, but can still progress swiftly to be a medical
emergency.

THE TUMBLER TEST

Press the side of a tumbler (a clear drinking glass) firmly against the child's
skin. (It's probably much harder to see a rash on darker skin, but you can check
any lighter areas such as the palms and soles of the feet.) If you can still see the
rash through the glass, the baby or toddler is very likely to have septicaemia.
Go to A&E or call an ambulance immediately.

By droplets from the throat, sneezes, hand contact etc

What to do: emergency action
If you suspect bacterial meningitis or viral meningitis it must be treated as a medical emergency. Go straight to the emergency (A&E) department of your local hospital no matter what time of the day or night. If you are not near a hospital call an ambulance on 999 or NHS Direct (0845 4647), who may ask you to take the "tumbler" (or glass) test if a rash has appeared.

Treatment
In hospital, staff will test for the disease using blood tests, a CT scan and a sample of spinal fluid taken from the patient. Bacterial meningitis will probably be treated in an intensive care unit (ICU) with steroids and antibiotics. Viral meningitis may not need hospital treatment, just rest and recuperation for up to two weeks. Severe cases of viral meningitis may need similiar treatment to that for bacterial meningitis.

Possible side effects of the vaccine
Injection site inflammation, temporary crankiness in babies.

Why we need the vaccine
Four vaccines – namely the MMR, Meningitis C, Pneumococcal and the DTaP/IPV/Hib vaccination – provide some protection against the majority of likely bacterial or viral cases of meningitis. Before the introduction of the vaccine in 1999 the type C strain accounted for around forty percent of meningococcal cases in the UK.

Alternative to the vaccine that would guarantee safety from infection
None. A person exposed can take an antibiotic to reduce the chance of catching it.

Mumps

Symptoms and effects
Fever, headache, big puffed-out cheeks caused by infection of the saliva glands, shivering, avoiding light (it "hurts" the eyes) and "floppy" tiredness. Trouble or pain when swallowing (which you might just see as your child rejecting food and drink if they're too little to tell you about the pain). Mumps can be very mild – it's believed one third of cases go unnoticed. But complications range from pancreatitis to viral meningitis. Rarer side effects include deafness; brain inflammation in one out of 5000 kids.

How it can be spread
Airborne drops in sneezes, coughs, caused by a virus.

Treatment
At home, you can wait out the week and try painkillers and lots of fluids. Antibiotics won't help you get rid of the virus but see your doctor in case

complications are developing.

POSSIBLE SIDE EFFECTS OF THE VACCINE

Low-grade fever, which is related to the measles component, and in about one percent of cases slight facial swelling.

WHY WE NEED THE VACCINE

Before the MMR vaccine was introduced, about 1200 people a year in England and Wales went into hospital because of mumps.

ALTERNATIVE TO THE VACCINE THAT WOULD GUARANTEE SAFETY FROM INFECTION None.

Pertussis (whooping cough)

SYMPTOMS AND EFFECTS

An irritating cough and sniffly, cold-like symptoms usually develop within a week or two into distressing coughing fits and difficulty drawing breath after each set of coughing spasms. This can cause a distinctive "whooping" sound, but not always in small babies. The coughing often continues for two to three months. Sometimes vomiting occurs. More rarely it can cause convulsions and coma, and death which is more likely to happen in babies under 1 year old; survivors may have permanent lung or brain damage.

HOW IT CAN BE SPREAD

Coughs, sneezes, contact with bacteria on hand, tissue etc. The bacteria is highly contagious – three vaccine doses by the age of 6 months are needed to give high protection to a baby.

TREATMENT

Antibiotics may be prescribed if it's diagnosed early (the first few weeks). Because babies under 1 are so vulnerable to whooping cough, they may need treatment including oxygen in hospital. Older children may need the usual home flu remedies of lots of cuddles and fluids.

POSSIBLE SIDE EFFECTS OF THE VACCINE

The modern vaccine causes far fewer side effects than the old one. Possible sore arm from jab and, rarely, low-grade fever, irritability, redness at jab site, brief fit in the 24 hours afterwards, with no long-term effects. The vaccine lasts about five to ten years.

WHY WE NEED THE VACCINE

Whooping cough, before there was a vaccine, killed thousands of children, especially smaller and more vulnerable babies. More than half of babies under 1 with the illness are hospitalised. Even if it is not fatal, the illness is very distressing and frightening for babies and their parents.

ALTERNATIVE TO THE VACCINE THAT WOULD GUARANTEE SAFETY FROM INFECTION None.

Pneumococcal infection

SYMPTOMS AND EFFECTS

Fever, fussiness or listlessness, sensitivity to bright light, headache. If these symptoms are accompanied by a distinctive red or purple rash and neck stiffness, it could mean meningitis (see p. 44) and/or blood poisoning. Pneumococcal infection can also damage the lungs and cause pneumonia.

HOW IT CAN BE SPREAD

Sneezes, coughs, dribble. From contact with the bacteria to symptoms may be less than 24 hours.

TREATMENT

Usually emergency hospital treatment with antibiotics.

POSSIBLE SIDE EFFECTS OF THE VACCINE

Rarely, fever, redness at the jab site. Even more rarely, vomiting or diarrhoea.

WHY WE NEED THE VACCINE

Pneumococcal disease results in serious infections of lungs, blood and ears and is a major cause of meningitis in kids (mostly under 2). The vaccine stops the seven types of bacteria that cause most cases here.

ALTERNATIVE TO THE VACCINE THAT WOULD GUARANTEE SAFETY FROM INFECTION None.

Poliomyelitis (infant paralysis, "Polio")

SYMPTOMS AND EFFECTS

Nausea, diarrhoea, fever, vomiting, muscle stiffness, nerve damage, five per-cent who get it will die from their breathing muscles being paralysed and half of the survivors will have permanent paralysis of the legs.

HOW IT CAN BE SPREAD

A virus spread by saliva and poo (for example, due to a nappy-changing hygiene problem).

TREATMENT

Polio is incurable though efforts can be made to alleviate the symptoms, hasten recovery and avert complications. The leg paralysis caused by polio may be temporary, improve very gradually over many years, or permanent. Children under 5 are more likely to have permanent paralysis of one leg while older kids up to the age of 15 are more likely to have it in both legs.

POSSIBLE SIDE EFFECTS OF THE VACCINE

See "Pertussis" (opposite). (It's usually given together with pertussis and tetanus.)

WHY WE NEED THE VACCINE

While many people believe polio has been eradicated, in fact it is still a serious problem in many places in the world, including India. Without immunisation, another outbreak of polio here and elsewhere would be inevitable. Polio, like other diseases, doesn't respect borders or need a passport.

ALTERNATIVE TO THE VACCINE THAT WOULD GUARANTEE SAFETY FROM INFECTION None.

Rubella (German measles)

SYMPTOMS AND EFFECTS

Swollen glands around the neck, groin and/or armpits, a pinky-to-red rash on the head and neck behind the ears for two to three days, slight fever, joint pain in adults (it is useful to diagnose all the family). Rubella varies in its effects. It can be devastating. If transmitted to an unimmunised pregnant woman in the first eight to ten weeks of pregnancy, there's a ninety percent chance it will cause severe birth defects, including blindness, deafness, mental retardation; the risk continues to twenty weeks of pregnancy. Symptoms can last two to three weeks. A person with rubella is contagious for a week before the rash appears and until five days after it first appears. A person who knows they have rubella must stay home until after the contagious period to avoid passing it to a pregnant woman at risk.

HOW IT CAN BE SPREAD

Very contagious: coughs and sneezes caused by a virus. It is contagious for about a week before the rash appears.

TREATMENT

Stay home and don't go to the doctor if you think your child has it as the risks of passing it to a pregnant woman are too high. Call your GP or NHS Direct (0845 4647) for advice. Treatment at home: as for measles, but you must avoid contact with others due to the risk.

POSSIBLE SIDE EFFECTS OF THE VACCINE

Slight fever and sore arm are the most common; some women develop transient joint pain.

WHY WE NEED THE VACCINE

Before immunisation it was a very common cause of deafness.

ALTERNATIVE TO THE VACCINE THAT WOULD GUARANTEE SAFETY FROM INFECTION None. Women need to be immunised up to one month before getting pregnant.

Tetanus

SYMPTOMS AND EFFECTS

Muscle spasms, stiff jaw and neck, breathing problems, convulsions, the nervous system shuts down, often leads to death.

HOW IT CAN BE SPREAD

A common microorganism in dirt and manure, which will produce a toxin (poison) if it gets into a deep cut or puncture wound. The bacteria that causes the disease can't be taken out of the environment so everyone is at risk unless they've been immunised and had regular boosters.

TREATMENT

If you're not immunised against tetanus and you may have picked it up in a wound, you'll need a special tetanus immunoglobulin dose (jab has side effects) *and* the vaccine.

POSSIBLE SIDE EFFECTS OF THE VACCINE

See "Pertussis" (p.46). (It's usually given in the same jab.)

WHY WE NEED THE VACCINE

Tetanus is rare in the UK and almost exclusively strikes older, under-vaccinated people. The death rate of patients is about ten percent. About 800,000 babies a year in developing countries die because of low or no vaccination.

ALTERNATIVE TO THE VACCINE THAT WOULD GUARANTEE SAFETY FROM INFECTION None.

NON-ROUTINE VACCINATIONS

Your child may need extra immunisation if they're seen to be at extra risk, for example because they may have had contact with tuberculosis or their mum has Hepatitis B. Aside from that, the only time you're likely to need extra vaccination is for travel to places considered "high-risk" for nasty diseases. Visit your doctor or a travel clinic a couple of months before your trip, so you'll be fully immune by the time you arrive. Children under 18 months are not usually given travel-related jabs but older kids generally have the same ones as adults. Doctors generally advise that babies who aren't immunised shouldn't go to high-risk areas. For health info on travel, including which jabs you'll need, visit www.fitfortravel.nhs.uk.

Part 4: More info & Contacts

MENINGITIS/MENINGOCOCCAL

These websites and helplines offer more info on the signs and symptoms of meningitis and blood poisoning caused by meningococcal and other bacteria, as well as information for families affected by meningitis.

www.meningitis-trust.org

For symptom worries: 24- hour phone line 0800 028 18 28
The Meningitis Trust is a UK charity providing practical help and support to families who have experienced meningitis, and working to raise awareness of the illness and its symptoms and treatment.

www.meningitis.org

For symptom worries: 24- hour phone line 080 8800 3344
The Meningitis Research Foundation is another group which raises awareness and promotes research into meningitis and septicaemia. Lots of info on the site, including FAQs.

GENERAL CHILD HEALTH

None of the following handy reference books and websites should be considered a substitute for individual, face-to-face medical diagnosis and advice. As with all books that involve medical information, get the latest edition. Don't forget to check for these at your local library if they're too expensive for your budget. Also make sure any website you get info from is a large mainstream site that's regularly updated with all the latest medical news.

WEBSITES

www.nhs.uk

Now rebranded as "NHS Your health, your choices" the NHS portal page has masses of relevant information on all aspects of health care. Bookmark this one.

www.nhsdirect.nhs.uk

Phone line 0845 4647

Contact the nurse-led phone line for information or queries on all child health matters. The website has self-help information too.

www.nhs.uk/planners/birthtofive/Pages/BirthtoFive.aspx

Basic guidance from the NHS on various baby essentials, health and development and other key issues for parents.

www.nctpregnancyandbabycare.com

Enquiry line 0300 33 00 770 (Mon – Thurs 9am – 5pm, Fri 9am – 4pm) The NCT (National Childbirth Trust) is the UK's leading charity supporting parents through pregnancy and the early weeks with a baby. Nationwide network of branches run courses for new parents to help them learn how to look after their baby.

www.bbc.co.uk/health

This is an excellent general health website with plenty of advice relating to young children, and a good section on asthma.

www.ich.ucl.ac.uk

The joint website of the Great Ormond Street Hospital and the Institute of Child Health, University College London, includes factsheets on various common childhood health problems, handy hints on bringing a child to hospital, a round up of support groups for families with kids who have certain conditions, advice from child health experts (including an alphabetical archive of

"Dr Jane's" down-to-earth advice on everything from pigeon toes to hayfever) and a glossary of terms you may need to understand.

BOOKS

When Your Child is Ill: A Home Guide for Parents (BMA Family Doctor)
by H.B. Valman, Dorling Kindersley, 2008
This is the "official" British Medical Association book on how to manage your sick child. Very easy to use and well illustrated. It has a great development chart and some useful but rather graphic photos of disgustingly erupting things you'd normally not want to see unless there are some already on your kid and you need to know what they are. Contains everything from limping and sniffles to whooping cough and muscular dystrophy. It also includes rudimentary first aid and has sensible flow charts that direct you to the right treatment.

Baby and Child Healthcare: The Essential A-Z Home Reference to Children's Illnesses, Symptoms and Treatments
by Miriam Stoppard, Dorling Kindersley, 2001
Dr Stoppard has written a whole string of books on baby and child care, so if you like her style, this is the one for you.

Natural Health for Kids: How to Give Your Child the Very Best Start in Life
by John Briffa, Penguin, 2007
Comprehensive and accessible "natural" health care guide for common childhood conditions such as asthma, allergies, bee stings and the dreaded nits. Remember to have a diagnosis confirmed by a doctor, and consider the doctor's advice, before treating with a natural remedy.

Natural Health for Kids: Complementary Treatments for More than 50 Ailments
by Sarah Wilson, Hamlyn, 2006
Draws on a range of holistic therapies such as aromatherapy, reflexology, herbalism and nutritional therapy to treat minor ailments and maintain good health. Again, get a medical diagnosis and advice before proceeding.

IMMUNISATION/VACCINATION

You should know that many anti-vaccination websites and books have authoritative-sounding titles which make them sound "official". And that "reviews" on sites such as Amazon praising them to the skies and saying they're "backed up" or "with medical facts" are not necessarily reliable. (Lynne McTaggart, author of the *Vaccination Bible* has also written a book on how the power of the mind can change the bacterial content of water, believes in faith healing and conducts "experiments" to try to prove that "thought intentions" sent by people concentrating can lower the crime rate in another country.) Also, be aware when reading American books (such as *The Vaccine Book* by Dr William Sears) or info on US sites that there is a different immunisation schedule for kids over there and different vaccines, and the information can be entirely irrelevant to the medical situation here in the UK. Here are some recommended useful sites.

WEBSITES

www.immunisation.nhs.uk
The best "official" website about all aspects of immunisation. You can download a childhood immunisation schedule, and there is clear detail about diseases and their vaccinations, lists of frequently

asked questions and all the latest research on MMR and its safety.

www.dh.gov.uk

The Department of Health's site has a downloadable copy of the "Green Book", the professional bible of UK immunisation (click on Public Health, then Health Protection, then Immunisation), but it's massive and cannot be updated as fast as the immunisation website (above) can. This one's useful if you want incredibly detailed info on a specific aspect of immunisation or a particular disease and treatment. Click on "Yellow Book" for travel vaccination info.

www.path.org

View the key achievements of the children's vaccine programme worldwide. The Vaccine Resource Library looks at the arguments surrounding immunisation and gives guidance on diseases.

www.who.int

From the home page of the World Health Organization, search "Disease outbreak news" to see where diseases on the UK immunisation schedule pop up elsewhere in the world, or search "immunisation programme" to see the work still going on to combat global diseases.

www.polioeradication.org

This is the website of the Global Polio Eradication Initiative. The website has factsheets and answers to the most frequently asked questions about polio, as well as moving photographs, important stories and hornswoggling statistics.

www.briandeer.com/wakefield-deer.htm

A respected British investigative reporter wraps up the Dr Wakefield anti-MMR campaign story.

www.badscience.net

A British journo and doctor, Ben Goldacre runs a funny and entertaining site while he's being serious about why homeopathy won't work any better than a sugar pill, how the anti-MMR rumours gained such a following despite being utterly wrong, and how hopeless most reporters and TV shows are when explaining science.

BOOKS

Autism's False Prophets: Bad Science, Risky Medicine and the Search for the Cure
by Paul Offit, Columbia University Press, 2008
The evidence is now in, and clearly explained here. These things do not cause autism: the measles mumps rubella (MMR) vaccine, other childhood vaccines, and mercury. This is a careful, clear and fair explanation of why people were led so badly astray. Dr Offit is head of infectious diseases and director of the Vaccine Education Centre at the well-respected Children's Hospital of Philadelphia in the USA, and all profits from this book go to medical research into autism.

Bad Science
by Ben Goldacre, Harper Perennial UK
The book which matches the website (see above).

Vaccine: The Controversial Story of Medicine's Greatest Lifesaver
by Arthur Allen, Norton, 2007
Mr Allen uses his long experience as a journalist to detail the history of vaccines including a clear-eyed cataloguing of the problems, and covers the fight against polio, the eradication of smallpox , the anti-vaccination movement and the autism controversy.